ADHD & ASD Parenting Journal

Alison M Thompson

Copyright © 2020 Alison M Thompson

All rights reserved. This book or any portion thereof may not be reproduced or used in any manner whatsoever without the express written permission of the publisher.

First Printing 2020

ISBN 9781661225810

Published by ADHD Kids: www.adhdkids.org.uk

How To Use This Journal

The ADHD & ASD Parenting Journal has been specially designed to help you keep a record of your child's behaviour quickly and easily. The journal lasts three months and is an ideal way for you to monitor your child's progress, identify useful strategies and provide your paediatrician with a record of your child's ADHD or ASD.

On the first two pages you can note down useful details about your child, and target behaviours to manage. This section will be particularly useful for anyone outside the immediate family who may care for your child – babysitters, childminders, family, friends, teachers – as it gives them a snapshot of your child.

The following pages are two-page daily spreads with sections for food and sleep, medication, incidents and strategies, and appointments, plus space for you to add any other information. There's even a section for your child's teacher to complete, if you want to share the journal with school.

Each spread is undated, so you can start whenever you want. Simply add the date and circle the day of the week – this is really important, as it will make it easier for you to spot behaviour patterns. You can also "grade" how each part of the day has gone by circling one of the smiley faces. Page numbers make it easy to find specific days.

The front cover has a space where you can add your child's name in marker pen. This is really useful if you have more than one child with SEN and want to keep a journal for each, or if you are sending the journal into school.

Finally, at the end of the book there are some blank pages for notes.

I hope you find this journal useful. If you have any feedback or comments please let me know, I'd love to hear from you! You can email me at alison@adhdkids.org.uk

If you'd like more information about ADHD, have a look at:

My website: www.adhdkids.org.uk

The ADHD Kids Online Parenting Programme: www.adhdkidsonline.com

My book, "The Boy From Hell: Life with a Child with ADHD" by Alison M Thompson, available on Amazon.

Good luck!

Alison x

CHILD'S NAME	Deanna Girdlestone

EMERGENCY CONTACT DETAILS
07572464199 (mum).

ALLERGIES / FOODS TO AVOID
None

MEDICATION
Melatonin. etc.

LIKES	DISLIKES
Music Clothes Makeup. Animals	Does not like change. Not doing as told

BEHAVIOURS TO REWARD

Going to bed.
breakfast.
Doing as told.

BEHAVIOURS TO IGNORE

Winging to get attention.

BEHAVIOURS WITH CONSEQUENCES

Swearing,
Kicking
Pinching.

| DATE 1/2/11/2022 | M (T) W T F S S |

SLEEP 9pm   Notes
Woke at: 11.30pm, 1.30 AM, 2.30 AM
Bed at: 9pm.

BREAKFAST
Nothing refused

DINNER
Nuggets e chips.

LUNCH
Lettuce
Sandwich
Crisps
Juice. G

SNACKS
Grapes.

MEDICATION & EFFECTS
Melatonin x2.

INCIDENTS

What happened?	Trigger(s)	Actions / Results
Mum worked till 11pm Screaming e throwing things Hitting dad.	Mummy working	

APPOINTMENTS

MORNING ☺ 😐 ☹(circled)

Did not go to school on 2/11/22. Was very tired, eyes swollen, distressed.

AFTERNOON ☺(circled) 😐 ☹

Happy but tired

EVENING ☺ 😐(circled) ☹

Very tired.

SCHOOL ☺ 😐 ☹(circled)

Did not attend.

DATE	3/11/22	M T W (T) F S S

SLEEP
Woke at:
Bed at:

Notes

BREAKFAST	cereal with milk	DINNER	Sausage & chips beans.
LUNCH	lettuce Sam crisps Juice	SNACKS	Banana

MEDICATION & EFFECTS

INCIDENTS

What happened?	Trigger(s)	Actions / Results
Fighting, biting refused to get dressed	mams	Put in car with clothes got dressed Went to school.

APPOINTMENTS

MORNING 🙂 😐 ☹(circled) Did not want to go as worried about maths. Teacher greeted her at office she went in.

AFTERNOON 🙂(circled) 😐 ☹ Good afternoon at school.

EVENING 🙂(circled) 😐 ☹ tired long day at school

SCHOOL 🙂 😐 ☹(circled) tired

| DATE 4/5/11 | M T W T F (S) S |

| SLEEP 10.15 | Notes |
| Woke at: 1-15, 2.30pm. |
| Bed at: 9.30. |

| BREAKFAST Nothing | DINNER Pizza |
| LUNCH Pasta | SNACKS Crisps. |

MEDICATION & EFFECTS

INCIDENTS

What happened?	Trigger(s)	Actions / Results
Hitting/ brother/ Kicking Swearing	Brothers Birthday.	

APPOINTMENTS

MORNING ☺ 😐 ☹(circled) Did not want to go to school

AFTERNOON ☺(circled) 😐 ☹

EVENING ☺ 😐 ☹(circled) Was sick after eating pizza.

SCHOOL ☺ 😐 ☹

| DATE | 12/11/22 | M T W T F (S) S |

SLEEP
Woke at: 7·30 Am
Bed at: 9·30 Am

Notes

| BREAKFAST Pancakes. | DINNER |
| LUNCH | SNACKS |

MEDICATION & EFFECTS

INCIDENTS

| What happened? | Trigger(s) | Actions / Results |
| We took Facebook off her phone put Parental contras on | no facebook | Phone removed. |

APPOINTMENTS

MORNING ☺ ☹ (☹) Bad morning

AFTERNOON (☺) ☹ ☹ Happy Getting ready for party.

EVENING ☺ ☹ (☹) Very tired by 10pm

SCHOOL ☺ ☹ ☹

| DATE | 13/12/22 | M T W T F S (S) |

SLEEP HAD A friend **Notes** Stay over.
Woke at: 5AM
Bed at: 12PM   PARTY.

BREAKFAST toast butter

DINNER turkey unicorns with potatoes.

LUNCH

SNACKS yogurts.

MEDICATION & EFFECTS

INCIDENTS

What happened?
Cried
Swear
hit &
Scream

Trigger(s)
tired.

Actions / Results
Fell
asleep
3 hours.

APPOINTMENTS

MORNING 🙂 ☹️(circled) ☹️ — tired did not sleep to well friend stayed.

AFTERNOON 🙂 😐 ☹️(circled) — Very grumpy Swearing & Screaming fell asleep at 3pm - 6pm

EVENING 🙂(circled) 😐 ☹️ — She was ok.

SCHOOL 🙂 😐 ☹️

DATE	14/11/22	**M** T W T F S S

SLEEP
Woke at: 7AM
Bed at: 9pm.

Notes

BREAKFAST Chips & Bacon roll	DINNER Beans & fish cakes.
LUNCH Jam Sand.	SNACKS Pot noodle.

MEDICATION & EFFECTS

INCIDENTS

What happened?	Trigger(s)	Actions / Results
Dad put Parental controls on phone Sat. Caused a two hour meltdown		as she wanted it max.

APPOINTMENTS

MORNING 🙂 😐 ☹️ not happy as I had taken brother to hospital spoken to her on the phone. afte she was fine

AFTERNOON 🙂 😐 (☹️)

EVENING (🙂) 😐 ☹️ Hot Bath

SCHOOL 🙂 😐 ☹️ no school

DATE	15/11	M **T** W T F S S

SLEEP
Woke at: 7AM
Bed at: 9PM

Notes
Woke x2
In the early hours

BREAKFAST
toast

DINNER
fishcakes/
Alphabites.

LUNCH
Sandwiches
Jelly, crisps

SNACKS
Grapes.

MEDICATION & EFFECTS

INCIDENTS

What happened?	Trigger(s)	Actions / Results

APPOINTMENTS

MORNING ☺ 😐 ☹

Called me a C____ because hair was not right.

AFTERNOON ☺ 😐 ☹

EVENING ☺ 😐 ☹

Complained of stomach pain had upset stomach.

SCHOOL ☺ 😐 ☹

Not good. Two friends not being nice to her.

DATE	16 / 11	M T (W) T F S S

SLEEP
Woke at: 7AM
Bed at: 9PM

Notes: Woke up twice.

BREAKFAST
Toast
Duece/

DINNER Pasta

LUNCH Pasta

SNACKS Crisps.

MEDICATION & EFFECTS

INCIDENTS

What happened?	Trigger(s)	Actions / Results
Major melt down kicked me. and threw it over the floor.	Bubble tea not tasting nice.	Put it in the bin

APPOINTMENTS

MORNING ☺ 😐 ☹

AFTERNOON ☺ 😐 ☹

Bubble tea - got called names again!!

EVENING ☺ 😐 ☹

Did not make it to gymnastics as I could not sit in hall with her. Kicked car and screamed and started swearing.

SCHOOL ☺ 😐 ☹

DATE	17/11	M T W **T** F S S

SLEEP   Notes
Woke at: 2.30 AM - 4.45 AM 7PM.
Bed at: 9 PM

BREAKFAST	DINNER
Toast.	Fish cakes & waffles.

LUNCH	SNACKS
Sandwiches Crisps Juice	Grapes.

MEDICATION & EFFECTS

INCIDENTS

What happened?	Trigger(s)	Actions / Results
Hair, not right. Fallen out with friend at school	Melt down because hair was sticking up. Got to school started screaming	

APPOINTMENTS

MORNING ☺ 😐 ☹(circled)

HAIR, FALL OUT WITH friend, Got to gates screamed non stop.

AFTERNOON ☺(circled) 😐 ☹

Good day at school.

EVENING ☺(circled) 😐 ☹

OK.

SCHOOL ☺(circled) 😐 ☹

OK.

DATE	18/11	M T W T (F) S S

SLEEP
Woke at: 2.30, 5.00 AM 7pm.
Bed at:

Notes

BREAKFAST	toast	DINNER	Chicken strips chips.
LUNCH	fish finger chips & Beans	SNACKS	

MEDICATION & EFFECTS

INCIDENTS

What happened?	Trigger(s)	Actions / Results
Scream, Swear, Shouting, Calling names, throwing things.	What clothes to wear for mufti Day. Mummy went out with friends	Went to school in first set of clothes. Went out came back hour later

APPOINTMENTS

MORNING 🙂 😐 ☹️ (😐 circled)

4 different outfits could not decide what to where.

AFTERNOON 🙂 😐 ☹️ (🙂 circled)

Dance lessons after school really enjoyed it.

EVENING 🙂 😐 ☹️ (😐 circled)

Meltdown mommy went out with friends, for one hour had to come home.

SCHOOL 🙂 😐 ☹️ (🙂 circled)

DATE	M T W T F S S

SLEEP

Woke at:

Bed at:

Notes

BREAKFAST	DINNER
LUNCH	SNACKS

MEDICATION & EFFECTS

INCIDENTS

What happened?	Trigger(s)	Actions / Results

APPOINTMENTS

MORNING ☺ 😐 ☹

AFTERNOON ☺ 😐 ☹

EVENING ☺ 😐 ☹

SCHOOL ☺ 😐 ☹

DATE	M T W T F S S

SLEEP

Woke at:

Bed at:

Notes

BREAKFAST	DINNER
LUNCH	SNACKS

MEDICATION & EFFECTS

INCIDENTS

What happened?	Trigger(s)	Actions / Results

APPOINTMENTS

MORNING ☺ 😐 ☹

AFTERNOON ☺ 😐 ☹

EVENING ☺ 😐 ☹

SCHOOL ☺ 😐 ☹

DATE	M T W T F S S

SLEEP Notes

Woke at:

Bed at:

BREAKFAST	DINNER
LUNCH	SNACKS

MEDICATION & EFFECTS

INCIDENTS

What happened?	Trigger(s)	Actions / Results

APPOINTMENTS

MORNING ☺ 😐 ☹

AFTERNOON ☺ 😐 ☹

EVENING ☺ 😐 ☹

SCHOOL ☺ 😐 ☹

DATE	M T W T F S S

SLEEP   Notes

Woke at:

Bed at:

BREAKFAST	DINNER
LUNCH	SNACKS

MEDICATION & EFFECTS

INCIDENTS

What happened?	Trigger(s)	Actions / Results

APPOINTMENTS

MORNING ☺ 😐 ☹

AFTERNOON ☺ 😐 ☹

EVENING ☺ 😐 ☹

SCHOOL ☺ 😐 ☹

DATE	M T W T F S S

SLEEP　　　　　　Notes

Woke at:

Bed at:

BREAKFAST	DINNER
LUNCH	SNACKS

MEDICATION & EFFECTS

INCIDENTS

What happened?	Trigger(s)	Actions / Results

APPOINTMENTS

MORNING ☺ 😐 ☹

AFTERNOON ☺ 😐 ☹

EVENING ☺ 😐 ☹

SCHOOL ☺ 😐 ☹

DATE	M T W T F S S

SLEEP Notes

Woke at:

Bed at:

BREAKFAST	DINNER
LUNCH	SNACKS

MEDICATION & EFFECTS

INCIDENTS

What happened?	Trigger(s)	Actions / Results

APPOINTMENTS

MORNING ☺ 😐 ☹

AFTERNOON ☺ 😐 ☹

EVENING ☺ 😐 ☹

SCHOOL ☺ 😐 ☹

DATE	M T W T F S S

SLEEP Notes

Woke at:

Bed at:

BREAKFAST	DINNER
LUNCH	SNACKS

MEDICATION & EFFECTS

INCIDENTS

What happened?	Trigger(s)	Actions / Results

APPOINTMENTS

MORNING ☺ 😐 ☹

AFTERNOON ☺ 😐 ☹

EVENING ☺ 😐 ☹

SCHOOL ☺ 😐 ☹

DATE	M T W T F S S

SLEEP   Notes

Woke at:

Bed at:

BREAKFAST	DINNER
LUNCH	SNACKS

MEDICATION & EFFECTS

INCIDENTS

What happened?	Trigger(s)	Actions / Results

APPOINTMENTS

MORNING ☺ 😐 ☹

AFTERNOON ☺ 😐 ☹

EVENING ☺ 😐 ☹

SCHOOL ☺ 😐 ☹

DATE	M T W T F S S

SLEEP Notes

Woke at:

Bed at:

BREAKFAST	DINNER
LUNCH	SNACKS

MEDICATION & EFFECTS

INCIDENTS

What happened?	Trigger(s)	Actions / Results

APPOINTMENTS

MORNING ☺ 😐 ☹

AFTERNOON ☺ 😐 ☹

EVENING ☺ 😐 ☹

SCHOOL ☺ 😐 ☹

DATE	M T W T F S S

SLEEP Notes

Woke at:

Bed at:

BREAKFAST	DINNER
LUNCH	SNACKS

MEDICATION & EFFECTS

INCIDENTS		
What happened?	Trigger(s)	Actions / Results

APPOINTMENTS

MORNING ☺ 😐 ☹

AFTERNOON ☺ 😐 ☹

EVENING ☺ 😐 ☹

SCHOOL ☺ 😐 ☹

DATE	M T W T F S S

SLEEP   Notes

Woke at:

Bed at:

BREAKFAST	DINNER
LUNCH	SNACKS

MEDICATION & EFFECTS

INCIDENTS

What happened?	Trigger(s)	Actions / Results

APPOINTMENTS

MORNING ☺ 😐 ☹

AFTERNOON ☺ 😐 ☹

EVENING ☺ 😐 ☹

SCHOOL ☺ 😐 ☹

DATE	M T W T F S S

SLEEP Notes

Woke at:

Bed at:

BREAKFAST	DINNER
LUNCH	SNACKS

MEDICATION & EFFECTS

INCIDENTS		
What happened?	Trigger(s)	Actions / Results

APPOINTMENTS

MORNING 🙂 😐 ☹️

AFTERNOON 🙂 😐 ☹️

EVENING 🙂 😐 ☹️

SCHOOL 🙂 😐 ☹️

DATE	M T W T F S S

SLEEP Notes

Woke at:

Bed at:

BREAKFAST	DINNER
LUNCH	SNACKS

MEDICATION & EFFECTS

INCIDENTS

What happened?	Trigger(s)	Actions / Results

APPOINTMENTS

MORNING ☺ 😐 ☹

AFTERNOON ☺ 😐 ☹

EVENING ☺ 😐 ☹

SCHOOL ☺ 😐 ☹

DATE	M T W T F S S

SLEEP   Notes

Woke at:

Bed at:

BREAKFAST	DINNER
LUNCH	SNACKS

MEDICATION & EFFECTS

INCIDENTS

What happened?	Trigger(s)	Actions / Results

APPOINTMENTS

MORNING ☺ 😐 ☹

AFTERNOON ☺ 😐 ☹

EVENING ☺ 😐 ☹

SCHOOL ☺ 😐 ☹

| DATE | M T W T F S S |

SLEEP　　　　　Notes

Woke at:

Bed at:

BREAKFAST	DINNER
LUNCH	SNACKS

MEDICATION & EFFECTS

INCIDENTS

What happened?	Trigger(s)	Actions / Results

APPOINTMENTS

MORNING ☺ 😐 ☹

AFTERNOON ☺ 😐 ☹

EVENING ☺ 😐 ☹

SCHOOL ☺ 😐 ☹

| DATE | M T W T F S S |

SLEEP   Notes

Woke at:

Bed at:

BREAKFAST	DINNER
LUNCH	SNACKS

MEDICATION & EFFECTS

INCIDENTS

What happened?	Trigger(s)	Actions / Results

APPOINTMENTS

MORNING ☺ 😐 ☹

AFTERNOON ☺ 😐 ☹

EVENING ☺ 😐 ☹

SCHOOL ☺ 😐 ☹

DATE	M T W T F S S

SLEEP Notes

Woke at:

Bed at:

BREAKFAST	DINNER
LUNCH	SNACKS

MEDICATION & EFFECTS

INCIDENTS

What happened?	Trigger(s)	Actions / Results

APPOINTMENTS

MORNING ☺ 😐 ☹

AFTERNOON ☺ 😐 ☹

EVENING ☺ 😐 ☹

SCHOOL ☺ 😐 ☹

DATE	M T W T F S S

SLEEP   Notes

Woke at:

Bed at:

BREAKFAST	DINNER
LUNCH	SNACKS

MEDICATION & EFFECTS

INCIDENTS

What happened?	Trigger(s)	Actions / Results

APPOINTMENTS

MORNING 🙂 😐 🙁

AFTERNOON 🙂 😐 🙁

EVENING 🙂 😐 🙁

SCHOOL 🙂 😐 🙁

DATE	M T W T F S S

SLEEP   Notes

Woke at:

Bed at:

BREAKFAST	DINNER
LUNCH	SNACKS

MEDICATION & EFFECTS

INCIDENTS

What happened?	Trigger(s)	Actions / Results

APPOINTMENTS

MORNING ☺ 😐 ☹

AFTERNOON ☺ 😐 ☹

EVENING ☺ 😐 ☹

SCHOOL ☺ 😐 ☹

DATE	M T W T F S S

SLEEP Notes

Woke at:

Bed at:

BREAKFAST	DINNER
LUNCH	SNACKS

MEDICATION & EFFECTS

INCIDENTS

What happened?	Trigger(s)	Actions / Results

APPOINTMENTS

MORNING ☺ 😐 ☹

AFTERNOON ☺ 😐 ☹

EVENING ☺ 😐 ☹

SCHOOL ☺ 😐 ☹

DATE	M T W T F S S

SLEEP　　　　　Notes

Woke at:

Bed at:

BREAKFAST	DINNER
LUNCH	SNACKS

MEDICATION & EFFECTS

INCIDENTS

What happened?	Trigger(s)	Actions / Results

APPOINTMENTS

MORNING ☺ 😐 ☹

AFTERNOON ☺ 😐 ☹

EVENING ☺ 😐 ☹

SCHOOL ☺ 😐 ☹

DATE	M T W T F S S

SLEEP   Notes

Woke at:

Bed at:

BREAKFAST	DINNER
LUNCH	SNACKS

MEDICATION & EFFECTS

INCIDENTS

What happened?	Trigger(s)	Actions / Results

APPOINTMENTS

MORNING ☺ 😐 ☹

AFTERNOON ☺ 😐 ☹

EVENING ☺ 😐 ☹

SCHOOL ☺ 😐 ☹

DATE	**M T W T F S S**

SLEEP Notes

Woke at:

Bed at:

BREAKFAST	DINNER
LUNCH	SNACKS

MEDICATION & EFFECTS

INCIDENTS

What happened?	Trigger(s)	Actions / Results

APPOINTMENTS

MORNING ☺ 😐 ☹

AFTERNOON ☺ 😐 ☹

EVENING ☺ 😐 ☹

SCHOOL ☺ 😐 ☹

DATE	M T W T F S S

SLEEP   Notes

Woke at:

Bed at:

BREAKFAST	DINNER
LUNCH	SNACKS

MEDICATION & EFFECTS

INCIDENTS

What happened?	Trigger(s)	Actions / Results

APPOINTMENTS

MORNING ☺ 😐 ☹

AFTERNOON ☺ 😐 ☹

EVENING ☺ 😐 ☹

SCHOOL ☺ 😐 ☹

DATE	M T W T F S S

SLEEP Notes

Woke at:

Bed at:

BREAKFAST	DINNER
LUNCH	SNACKS

MEDICATION & EFFECTS

INCIDENTS

What happened?	Trigger(s)	Actions / Results

APPOINTMENTS

MORNING ☺ 😐 ☹

AFTERNOON ☺ 😐 ☹

EVENING ☺ 😐 ☹

SCHOOL ☺ 😐 ☹

DATE	M T W T F S S

SLEEP Notes

Woke at:

Bed at:

BREAKFAST	DINNER
LUNCH	SNACKS

MEDICATION & EFFECTS

INCIDENTS

What happened?	Trigger(s)	Actions / Results

APPOINTMENTS

MORNING ☺ 😐 ☹

AFTERNOON ☺ 😐 ☹

EVENING ☺ 😐 ☹

SCHOOL ☺ 😐 ☹

DATE	M T W T F S S

SLEEP

Woke at:

Bed at:

Notes

BREAKFAST	DINNER
LUNCH	SNACKS

MEDICATION & EFFECTS

INCIDENTS

What happened?	Trigger(s)	Actions / Results

APPOINTMENTS

MORNING ☺ 😐 ☹

AFTERNOON ☺ 😐 ☹

EVENING ☺ 😐 ☹

SCHOOL ☺ 😐 ☹

DATE	M T W T F S S

SLEEP Notes

Woke at:

Bed at:

BREAKFAST	DINNER
LUNCH	SNACKS

MEDICATION & EFFECTS

INCIDENTS

What happened?	Trigger(s)	Actions / Results

APPOINTMENTS

MORNING ☺ 😐 ☹

AFTERNOON ☺ 😐 ☹

EVENING ☺ 😐 ☹

SCHOOL ☺ 😐 ☹

| DATE | M T W T F S S |

SLEEP Notes

Woke at:

Bed at:

BREAKFAST	DINNER
LUNCH	SNACKS

MEDICATION & EFFECTS

INCIDENTS

What happened?	Trigger(s)	Actions / Results

APPOINTMENTS

MORNING ☺ 😐 ☹

AFTERNOON ☺ 😐 ☹

EVENING ☺ 😐 ☹

SCHOOL ☺ 😐 ☹

DATE	M T W T F S S

SLEEP   Notes

Woke at:

Bed at:

BREAKFAST	DINNER
LUNCH	SNACKS

MEDICATION & EFFECTS

INCIDENTS

What happened?	Trigger(s)	Actions / Results

APPOINTMENTS

MORNING ☺ 😐 ☹

AFTERNOON ☺ 😐 ☹

EVENING ☺ 😐 ☹

SCHOOL ☺ 😐 ☹

DATE	M T W T F S S

SLEEP Notes

Woke at:

Bed at:

BREAKFAST	DINNER
LUNCH	SNACKS

MEDICATION & EFFECTS

INCIDENTS

What happened?	Trigger(s)	Actions / Results

APPOINTMENTS

MORNING ☺ 😐 ☹

AFTERNOON ☺ 😐 ☹

EVENING ☺ 😐 ☹

SCHOOL ☺ 😐 ☹

DATE	M T W T F S S

SLEEP
Woke at:

Bed at:

Notes

BREAKFAST	DINNER
LUNCH	SNACKS

MEDICATION & EFFECTS

INCIDENTS

What happened?	Trigger(s)	Actions / Results

APPOINTMENTS

MORNING ☺ 😐 ☹

AFTERNOON ☺ 😐 ☹

EVENING ☺ 😐 ☹

SCHOOL ☺ 😐 ☹

DATE	M T W T F S S

SLEEP Notes

Woke at:

Bed at:

BREAKFAST	DINNER
LUNCH	SNACKS

MEDICATION & EFFECTS

INCIDENTS

What happened?	Trigger(s)	Actions / Results

APPOINTMENTS

MORNING ☺ 😐 ☹

AFTERNOON ☺ 😐 ☹

EVENING ☺ 😐 ☹

SCHOOL ☺ 😐 ☹

| DATE | M T W T F S S |

SLEEP Notes

Woke at:

Bed at:

BREAKFAST	DINNER
LUNCH	SNACKS

MEDICATION & EFFECTS

INCIDENTS		
What happened?	Trigger(s)	Actions / Results

APPOINTMENTS

MORNING 🙂 😖 🙁

AFTERNOON 🙂 😖 🙁

EVENING 🙂 😖 🙁

SCHOOL 🙂 😖 🙁

DATE	M T W T F S S

SLEEP

Woke at:

Bed at:

Notes

BREAKFAST	DINNER
LUNCH	SNACKS

MEDICATION & EFFECTS

INCIDENTS

What happened?	Trigger(s)	Actions / Results

APPOINTMENTS

MORNING ☺ 😐 ☹

AFTERNOON ☺ 😐 ☹

EVENING ☺ 😐 ☹

SCHOOL ☺ 😐 ☹

DATE	M T W T F S S

SLEEP Notes

Woke at:

Bed at:

BREAKFAST	DINNER
LUNCH	SNACKS

MEDICATION & EFFECTS

INCIDENTS

What happened?	Trigger(s)	Actions / Results

APPOINTMENTS

MORNING ☺ 😐 ☹

AFTERNOON ☺ 😐 ☹

EVENING ☺ 😐 ☹

SCHOOL ☺ 😐 ☹

DATE	M T W T F S S

SLEEP

Woke at:

Bed at:

Notes

BREAKFAST	DINNER
LUNCH	SNACKS

MEDICATION & EFFECTS

INCIDENTS

What happened?	Trigger(s)	Actions / Results

APPOINTMENTS

MORNING 😊 😐 ☹️

AFTERNOON 😊 😐 ☹️

EVENING 😊 😐 ☹️

SCHOOL 😊 😐 ☹️

DATE	M T W T F S S

SLEEP Notes

Woke at:

Bed at:

BREAKFAST	DINNER
LUNCH	SNACKS

MEDICATION & EFFECTS

INCIDENTS

What happened?	Trigger(s)	Actions / Results

APPOINTMENTS

MORNING ☺ 😐 ☹

AFTERNOON ☺ 😐 ☹

EVENING ☺ 😐 ☹

SCHOOL ☺ 😐 ☹

DATE	M T W T F S S

SLEEP　　　　　Notes

Woke at:

Bed at:

BREAKFAST	DINNER
LUNCH	SNACKS

MEDICATION & EFFECTS

INCIDENTS

What happened?	Trigger(s)	Actions / Results

APPOINTMENTS

MORNING ☺ 😐 ☹

AFTERNOON ☺ 😐 ☹

EVENING ☺ 😐 ☹

SCHOOL ☺ 😐 ☹

DATE	M T W T F S S

SLEEP   Notes

Woke at:

Bed at:

BREAKFAST	DINNER
LUNCH	SNACKS

MEDICATION & EFFECTS

INCIDENTS

What happened?	Trigger(s)	Actions / Results

APPOINTMENTS

MORNING ☺ 😕 ☹

AFTERNOON ☺ 😕 ☹

EVENING ☺ 😕 ☹

SCHOOL ☺ 😕 ☹

DATE	M T W T F S S

SLEEP　　　　　Notes

Woke at:

Bed at:

BREAKFAST	DINNER
LUNCH	SNACKS

MEDICATION & EFFECTS

INCIDENTS

What happened?	Trigger(s)	Actions / Results

APPOINTMENTS

MORNING ☺ 😐 ☹

AFTERNOON ☺ 😐 ☹

EVENING ☺ 😐 ☹

SCHOOL ☺ 😐 ☹

DATE	M T W T F S S

SLEEP

Woke at:

Bed at:

Notes

BREAKFAST	DINNER
LUNCH	SNACKS

MEDICATION & EFFECTS

INCIDENTS

What happened?	Trigger(s)	Actions / Results

APPOINTMENTS

MORNING ☺ 😐 ☹

AFTERNOON ☺ 😐 ☹

EVENING ☺ 😐 ☹

SCHOOL ☺ 😐 ☹

DATE	M T W T F S S

SLEEP Notes
Woke at:
Bed at:

BREAKFAST	DINNER
LUNCH	SNACKS

MEDICATION & EFFECTS

INCIDENTS

What happened?	Trigger(s)	Actions / Results

APPOINTMENTS

MORNING ☺ 😐 ☹

AFTERNOON ☺ 😐 ☹

EVENING ☺ 😐 ☹

SCHOOL ☺ 😐 ☹

DATE	M T W T F S S

SLEEP　　　　Notes

Woke at:

Bed at:

BREAKFAST	DINNER
LUNCH	SNACKS

MEDICATION & EFFECTS

INCIDENTS

What happened?	Trigger(s)	Actions / Results

APPOINTMENTS

MORNING ☺ 😐 ☹

AFTERNOON ☺ 😐 ☹

EVENING ☺ 😐 ☹

SCHOOL ☺ 😐 ☹

DATE	M T W T F S S

SLEEP Notes

Woke at:

Bed at:

BREAKFAST	DINNER
LUNCH	SNACKS

MEDICATION & EFFECTS

INCIDENTS

What happened?	Trigger(s)	Actions / Results

APPOINTMENTS

MORNING ☺ 😐 ☹

AFTERNOON ☺ 😐 ☹

EVENING ☺ 😐 ☹

SCHOOL ☺ 😐 ☹

DATE	M T W T F S S

SLEEP

Woke at:

Bed at:

Notes

BREAKFAST	DINNER
LUNCH	SNACKS

MEDICATION & EFFECTS

INCIDENTS

What happened?	Trigger(s)	Actions / Results

APPOINTMENTS

MORNING ☺ 😐 ☹

AFTERNOON ☺ 😐 ☹

EVENING ☺ 😐 ☹

SCHOOL ☺ 😐 ☹

DATE	M T W T F S S

SLEEP Notes

Woke at:

Bed at:

BREAKFAST	DINNER
LUNCH	SNACKS

MEDICATION & EFFECTS

INCIDENTS

What happened?	Trigger(s)	Actions / Results

APPOINTMENTS

MORNING ☺ 😐 ☹

AFTERNOON ☺ 😐 ☹

EVENING ☺ 😐 ☹

SCHOOL ☺ 😐 ☹

DATE	M T W T F S S

SLEEP Notes

Woke at:

Bed at:

BREAKFAST	DINNER
LUNCH	SNACKS

MEDICATION & EFFECTS

INCIDENTS

What happened?	Trigger(s)	Actions / Results

APPOINTMENTS

MORNING ☺ 😐 ☹

AFTERNOON ☺ 😐 ☹

EVENING ☺ 😐 ☹

SCHOOL ☺ 😐 ☹

DATE	M T W T F S S

SLEEP Notes

Woke at:

Bed at:

BREAKFAST	DINNER
LUNCH	SNACKS

MEDICATION & EFFECTS

INCIDENTS

What happened?	Trigger(s)	Actions / Results

APPOINTMENTS

MORNING ☺ 😐 ☹

AFTERNOON ☺ 😐 ☹

EVENING ☺ 😐 ☹

SCHOOL ☺ 😐 ☹

DATE	M T W T F S S

SLEEP   Notes

Woke at:

Bed at:

BREAKFAST	DINNER
LUNCH	SNACKS

MEDICATION & EFFECTS

INCIDENTS

What happened?	Trigger(s)	Actions / Results

APPOINTMENTS

MORNING ☺ 😕 ☹

AFTERNOON ☺ 😕 ☹

EVENING ☺ 😕 ☹

SCHOOL ☺ 😕 ☹

DATE	M T W T F S S

SLEEP Notes

Woke at:

Bed at:

BREAKFAST	DINNER
LUNCH	SNACKS

MEDICATION & EFFECTS

INCIDENTS

What happened?	Trigger(s)	Actions / Results

APPOINTMENTS

MORNING ☺ 😐 ☹

AFTERNOON ☺ 😐 ☹

EVENING ☺ 😐 ☹

SCHOOL ☺ 😐 ☹

DATE	M T W T F S S

SLEEP   Notes

Woke at:

Bed at:

BREAKFAST	DINNER
LUNCH	SNACKS

MEDICATION & EFFECTS

INCIDENTS

What happened?	Trigger(s)	Actions / Results

APPOINTMENTS

MORNING ☺ 😐 ☹

AFTERNOON ☺ 😐 ☹

EVENING ☺ 😐 ☹

SCHOOL ☺ 😐 ☹

DATE	M T W T F S S

SLEEP

Woke at:

Bed at:

Notes

BREAKFAST	DINNER
LUNCH	SNACKS

MEDICATION & EFFECTS

INCIDENTS

What happened?	Trigger(s)	Actions / Results

APPOINTMENTS

MORNING ☺ 😕 ☹

AFTERNOON ☺ 😕 ☹

EVENING ☺ 😕 ☹

SCHOOL ☺ 😕 ☹

DATE	M T W T F S S

SLEEP Notes

Woke at:

Bed at:

BREAKFAST	DINNER
LUNCH	SNACKS

MEDICATION & EFFECTS

INCIDENTS

What happened?	Trigger(s)	Actions / Results

APPOINTMENTS

MORNING ☺ 😐 ☹

AFTERNOON ☺ 😐 ☹

EVENING ☺ 😐 ☹

SCHOOL ☺ 😐 ☹

DATE	M T W T F S S

SLEEP　　　　Notes

Woke at:

Bed at:

BREAKFAST	DINNER
LUNCH	SNACKS

MEDICATION & EFFECTS

INCIDENTS

What happened?	Trigger(s)	Actions / Results

APPOINTMENTS

MORNING ☺ 😐 ☹

AFTERNOON ☺ 😐 ☹

EVENING ☺ 😐 ☹

SCHOOL ☺ 😐 ☹

| DATE | M T W T F S S |

SLEEP

Woke at:

Bed at:

Notes

BREAKFAST	DINNER
LUNCH	SNACKS

MEDICATION & EFFECTS

INCIDENTS

What happened?	Trigger(s)	Actions / Results

APPOINTMENTS

MORNING ☺ 😐 ☹

AFTERNOON ☺ 😐 ☹

EVENING ☺ 😐 ☹

SCHOOL ☺ 😐 ☹

DATE	M T W T F S S

SLEEP   Notes

Woke at:

Bed at:

BREAKFAST	DINNER
LUNCH	SNACKS

MEDICATION & EFFECTS

INCIDENTS

What happened?	Trigger(s)	Actions / Results

APPOINTMENTS

MORNING ☺ 😐 ☹

AFTERNOON ☺ 😐 ☹

EVENING ☺ 😐 ☹

SCHOOL ☺ 😐 ☹

DATE	M T W T F S S

SLEEP Notes

Woke at:

Bed at:

BREAKFAST	DINNER
LUNCH	SNACKS

MEDICATION & EFFECTS

INCIDENTS		
What happened?	Trigger(s)	Actions / Results

APPOINTMENTS

MORNING ☺ 😐 ☹

AFTERNOON ☺ 😐 ☹

EVENING ☺ 😐 ☹

SCHOOL ☺ 😐 ☹

| DATE | M T W T F S S |

SLEEP Notes

Woke at:

Bed at:

BREAKFAST	DINNER
LUNCH	SNACKS

MEDICATION & EFFECTS

INCIDENTS

What happened?	Trigger(s)	Actions / Results

APPOINTMENTS

MORNING ☺ 😐 ☹

AFTERNOON ☺ 😐 ☹

EVENING ☺ 😐 ☹

SCHOOL ☺ 😐 ☹

DATE	M T W T F S S

SLEEP Notes
Woke at:
Bed at:

BREAKFAST	DINNER
LUNCH	SNACKS

MEDICATION & EFFECTS

INCIDENTS

What happened?	Trigger(s)	Actions / Results

APPOINTMENTS

MORNING ☺ 😕 ☹

AFTERNOON ☺ 😕 ☹

EVENING ☺ 😕 ☹

SCHOOL ☺ 😕 ☹

DATE	M T W T F S S

SLEEP Notes

Woke at:

Bed at:

BREAKFAST	DINNER
LUNCH	SNACKS

MEDICATION & EFFECTS

INCIDENTS

What happened?	Trigger(s)	Actions / Results

APPOINTMENTS

MORNING ☺ 😐 ☹

AFTERNOON ☺ 😐 ☹

EVENING ☺ 😐 ☹

SCHOOL ☺ 😐 ☹

DATE	M T W T F S S

SLEEP   Notes

Woke at:

Bed at:

BREAKFAST	DINNER
LUNCH	SNACKS

MEDICATION & EFFECTS

INCIDENTS

What happened?	Trigger(s)	Actions / Results

APPOINTMENTS

MORNING ☺ 😐 ☹

AFTERNOON ☺ 😐 ☹

EVENING ☺ 😐 ☹

SCHOOL ☺ 😐 ☹

DATE	M T W T F S S

SLEEP Notes

Woke at:

Bed at:

BREAKFAST	DINNER
LUNCH	SNACKS

MEDICATION & EFFECTS

INCIDENTS

What happened?	Trigger(s)	Actions / Results

APPOINTMENTS

MORNING ☺ 😐 ☹

AFTERNOON ☺ 😐 ☹

EVENING ☺ 😐 ☹

SCHOOL ☺ 😐 ☹

DATE	M T W T F S S

SLEEP Notes

Woke at:

Bed at:

BREAKFAST	DINNER
LUNCH	SNACKS

MEDICATION & EFFECTS

INCIDENTS

What happened?	Trigger(s)	Actions / Results

APPOINTMENTS

MORNING ☺ 😐 ☹

AFTERNOON ☺ 😐 ☹

EVENING ☺ 😐 ☹

SCHOOL ☺ 😐 ☹

DATE	M T W T F S S

SLEEP Notes

Woke at:

Bed at:

BREAKFAST	DINNER
LUNCH	SNACKS

MEDICATION & EFFECTS

INCIDENTS

What happened?	Trigger(s)	Actions / Results

APPOINTMENTS

MORNING ☺ 😐 ☹

AFTERNOON ☺ 😐 ☹

EVENING ☺ 😐 ☹

SCHOOL ☺ 😐 ☹

DATE	M T W T F S S

SLEEP Notes

Woke at:

Bed at:

BREAKFAST	DINNER
LUNCH	SNACKS

MEDICATION & EFFECTS

INCIDENTS

What happened?	Trigger(s)	Actions / Results

APPOINTMENTS

| MORNING ☺ 😐 ☹ |

| AFTERNOON ☺ 😐 ☹ |

| EVENING ☺ 😐 ☹ |

| SCHOOL ☺ 😐 ☹ |

DATE	M T W T F S S

SLEEP Notes

Woke at:

Bed at:

BREAKFAST	DINNER
LUNCH	SNACKS

MEDICATION & EFFECTS

INCIDENTS

What happened?	Trigger(s)	Actions / Results

APPOINTMENTS

MORNING ☺ 😐 ☹

AFTERNOON ☺ 😐 ☹

EVENING ☺ 😐 ☹

SCHOOL ☺ 😐 ☹

DATE	M T W T F S S

SLEEP   Notes

Woke at:

Bed at:

BREAKFAST	DINNER
LUNCH	SNACKS

MEDICATION & EFFECTS

INCIDENTS

What happened?	Trigger(s)	Actions / Results

APPOINTMENTS

MORNING ☺ 😐 ☹

AFTERNOON ☺ 😐 ☹

EVENING ☺ 😐 ☹

SCHOOL ☺ 😐 ☹

DATE	M T W T F S S

SLEEP Notes

Woke at:

Bed at:

BREAKFAST	DINNER
LUNCH	SNACKS

MEDICATION & EFFECTS

INCIDENTS

What happened?	Trigger(s)	Actions / Results

APPOINTMENTS

MORNING ☺ 😐 ☹

AFTERNOON ☺ 😐 ☹

EVENING ☺ 😐 ☹

SCHOOL ☺ 😐 ☹

DATE	M T W T F S S

SLEEP Notes

Woke at:

Bed at:

BREAKFAST	DINNER
LUNCH	SNACKS

MEDICATION & EFFECTS

INCIDENTS

What happened?	Trigger(s)	Actions / Results

APPOINTMENTS

MORNING ☺ 😐 ☹

AFTERNOON ☺ 😐 ☹

EVENING ☺ 😐 ☹

SCHOOL ☺ 😐 ☹

DATE	M T W T F S S

SLEEP　　　　Notes

Woke at:

Bed at:

BREAKFAST	DINNER

LUNCH	SNACKS

MEDICATION & EFFECTS

INCIDENTS

What happened?	Trigger(s)	Actions / Results

APPOINTMENTS

MORNING ☺ 😐 ☹

AFTERNOON ☺ 😐 ☹

EVENING ☺ 😐 ☹

SCHOOL ☺ 😐 ☹

DATE	M T W T F S S

SLEEP Notes

Woke at:

Bed at:

BREAKFAST	DINNER
LUNCH	SNACKS

MEDICATION & EFFECTS

INCIDENTS

What happened?	Trigger(s)	Actions / Results

APPOINTMENTS

MORNING ☺ 😐 ☹

AFTERNOON ☺ 😐 ☹

EVENING ☺ 😐 ☹

SCHOOL ☺ 😐 ☹

DATE	M T W T F S S

SLEEP   Notes

Woke at:

Bed at:

BREAKFAST	DINNER
LUNCH	SNACKS

MEDICATION & EFFECTS

INCIDENTS

What happened?	Trigger(s)	Actions / Results

APPOINTMENTS

MORNING ☺ 😐 ☹

AFTERNOON ☺ 😐 ☹

EVENING ☺ 😐 ☹

SCHOOL ☺ 😐 ☹

You're nearly at the end of the journal

...

Don't forget to order a new one

for the next three months

from Amazon

DATE	M T W T F S S

SLEEP

Woke at:

Bed at:

Notes

BREAKFAST	DINNER
LUNCH	SNACKS

MEDICATION & EFFECTS

INCIDENTS

What happened?	Trigger(s)	Actions / Results

APPOINTMENTS

MORNING ☺ 😐 ☹

AFTERNOON ☺ 😐 ☹

EVENING ☺ 😐 ☹

SCHOOL ☺ 😐 ☹

DATE	M T W T F S S

SLEEP　　　　Notes

Woke at:

Bed at:

BREAKFAST	DINNER
LUNCH	SNACKS

MEDICATION & EFFECTS

INCIDENTS

What happened?	Trigger(s)	Actions / Results

APPOINTMENTS

MORNING ☺ 😐 ☹

AFTERNOON ☺ 😐 ☹

EVENING ☺ 😐 ☹

SCHOOL ☺ 😐 ☹

DATE	M T W T F S S

SLEEP Notes

Woke at:

Bed at:

BREAKFAST	DINNER
LUNCH	SNACKS

MEDICATION & EFFECTS

INCIDENTS

What happened?	Trigger(s)	Actions / Results

APPOINTMENTS

MORNING ☺ 😐 ☹

AFTERNOON ☺ 😐 ☹

EVENING ☺ 😐 ☹

SCHOOL ☺ 😐 ☹

DATE	M T W T F S S

SLEEP Notes

Woke at:

Bed at:

BREAKFAST	DINNER
LUNCH	SNACKS

MEDICATION & EFFECTS

INCIDENTS

What happened?	Trigger(s)	Actions / Results

APPOINTMENTS

MORNING ☺ 😐 ☹

AFTERNOON ☺ 😐 ☹

EVENING ☺ 😐 ☹

SCHOOL ☺ 😐 ☹

DATE	M T W T F S S

SLEEP Notes

Woke at:

Bed at:

BREAKFAST	DINNER
LUNCH	SNACKS

MEDICATION & EFFECTS

INCIDENTS

What happened?	Trigger(s)	Actions / Results

APPOINTMENTS

MORNING ☺ 😐 ☹

AFTERNOON ☺ 😐 ☹

EVENING ☺ 😐 ☹

SCHOOL ☺ 😐 ☹

DATE	M T W T F S S

SLEEP Notes

Woke at:

Bed at:

BREAKFAST	DINNER
LUNCH	SNACKS

MEDICATION & EFFECTS

INCIDENTS

What happened?	Trigger(s)	Actions / Results

APPOINTMENTS

MORNING ☺ 😐 ☹

AFTERNOON ☺ 😐 ☹

EVENING ☺ 😐 ☹

SCHOOL ☺ 😐 ☹

DATE	M T W T F S S

SLEEP   Notes

Woke at:

Bed at:

BREAKFAST	DINNER
LUNCH	SNACKS

MEDICATION & EFFECTS

INCIDENTS

What happened?	Trigger(s)	Actions / Results

APPOINTMENTS

MORNING ☺ 😐 ☹

AFTERNOON ☺ 😐 ☹

EVENING ☺ 😐 ☹

SCHOOL ☺ 😐 ☹

| DATE | M T W T F S S |

SLEEP Notes

Woke at:

Bed at:

BREAKFAST	DINNER
LUNCH	SNACKS

MEDICATION & EFFECTS

INCIDENTS

What happened?	Trigger(s)	Actions / Results

APPOINTMENTS

MORNING ☺ 😐 ☹

AFTERNOON ☺ 😐 ☹

EVENING ☺ 😐 ☹

SCHOOL ☺ 😐 ☹

| DATE | M T W T F S S |

SLEEP　　　　　Notes

Woke at:

Bed at:

BREAKFAST	DINNER
LUNCH	SNACKS

MEDICATION & EFFECTS

INCIDENTS

What happened?	Trigger(s)	Actions / Results

APPOINTMENTS

MORNING ☺ 😐 ☹

AFTERNOON ☺ 😐 ☹

EVENING ☺ 😐 ☹

SCHOOL ☺ 😐 ☹

NOTES

NOTES

NOTES

Food.

Pot noodles.
butter

yogurt.
bread.
gammon

chicken.

fish cakes

fish fingers.
chips
Potato bites.
Brocoli
Yorkshire puddings
pork.
crisps
Nuts.

NOTES

NOTES

NOTES

NOTES

NOTES

NOTES

NOTES

Beef, Pork, Fish, beans.
low fat dairy.

Iron, omega 3, Zinc.
Tuna,
eggs.
Walnuts
Orange o r juice
Cherries
Cod.

5.69   17.99.
11.99   18.99
31.99.
12.79.
29.99.
18.90.
29.99.
18.99
13.00
22.00
13.99
19.99
7.99

Printed in Great Britain
by Amazon